Why Should I Get An Eye Exam?

A poetic eye care reminder for the entire family

Written by Kara Vance

Illustrated by TullipStudio

Dedication

To my children, who make me feel like a superwoman. Special shout out to my daughter, CiCi who listened to my first draft and said, "Mummy, you are a genius."

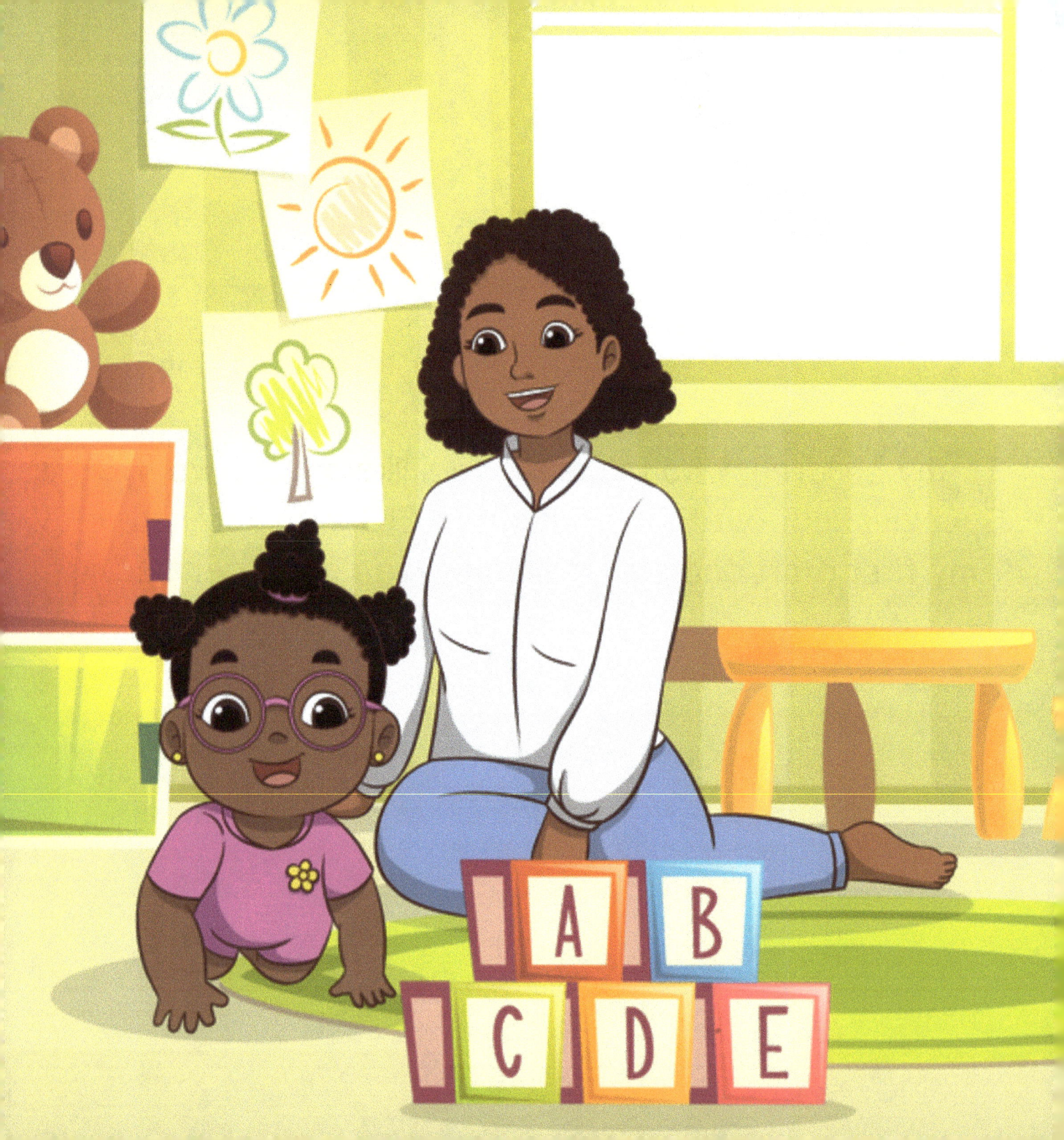

Why should I get an eye exam?
I can barely even crawl.

Your doctor might detect something
And help avoid close calls.

Why should I get an eye exam? Because my school says so?

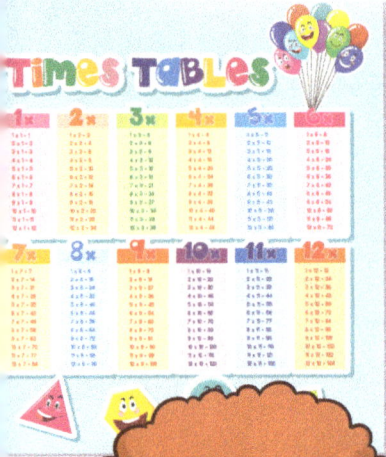

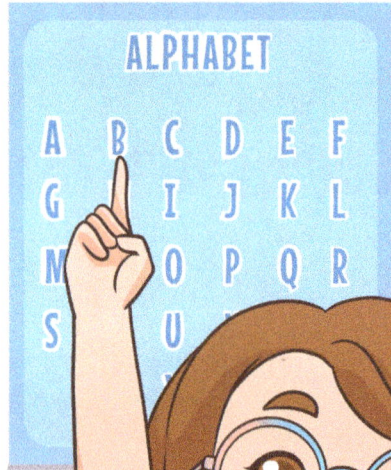

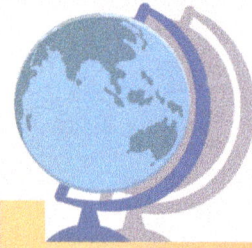

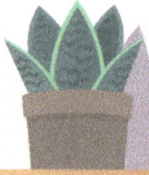

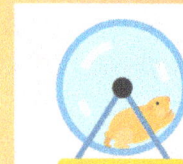

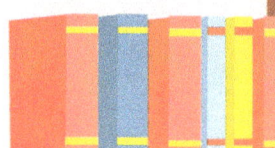

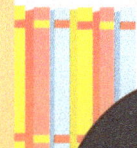

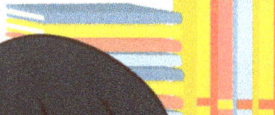

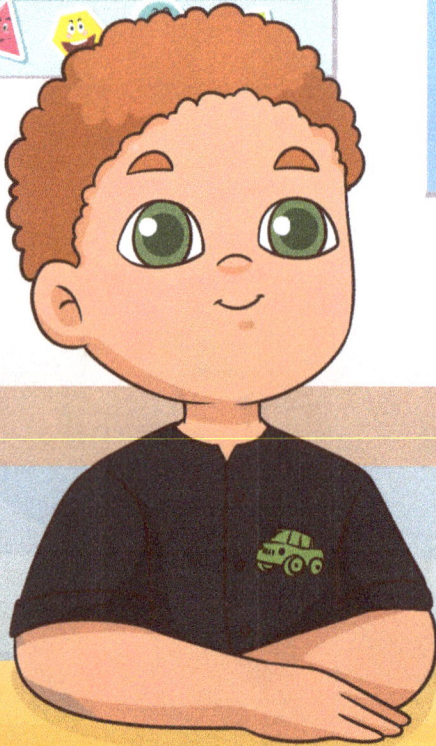

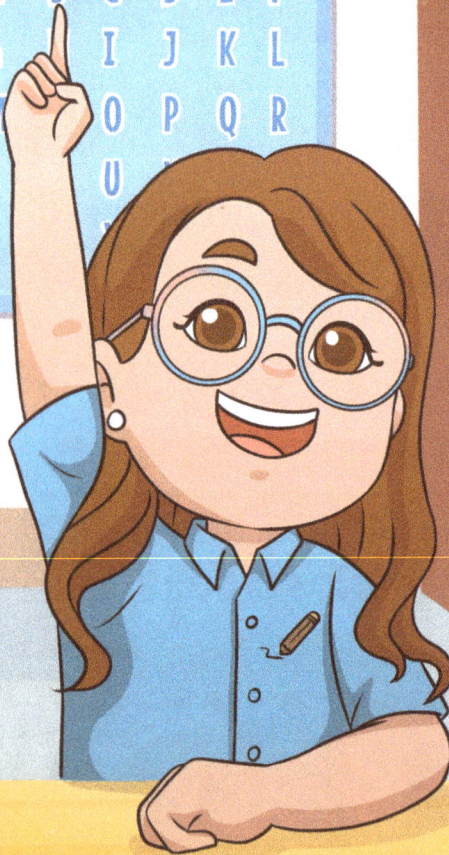

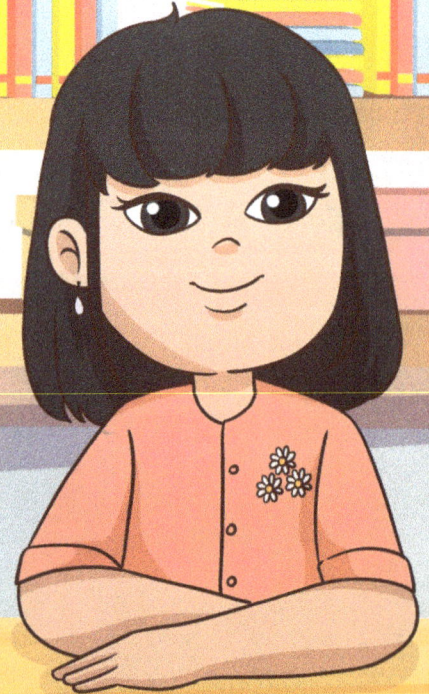

It's hard to learn when you can't see,
And vision changes as you grow.

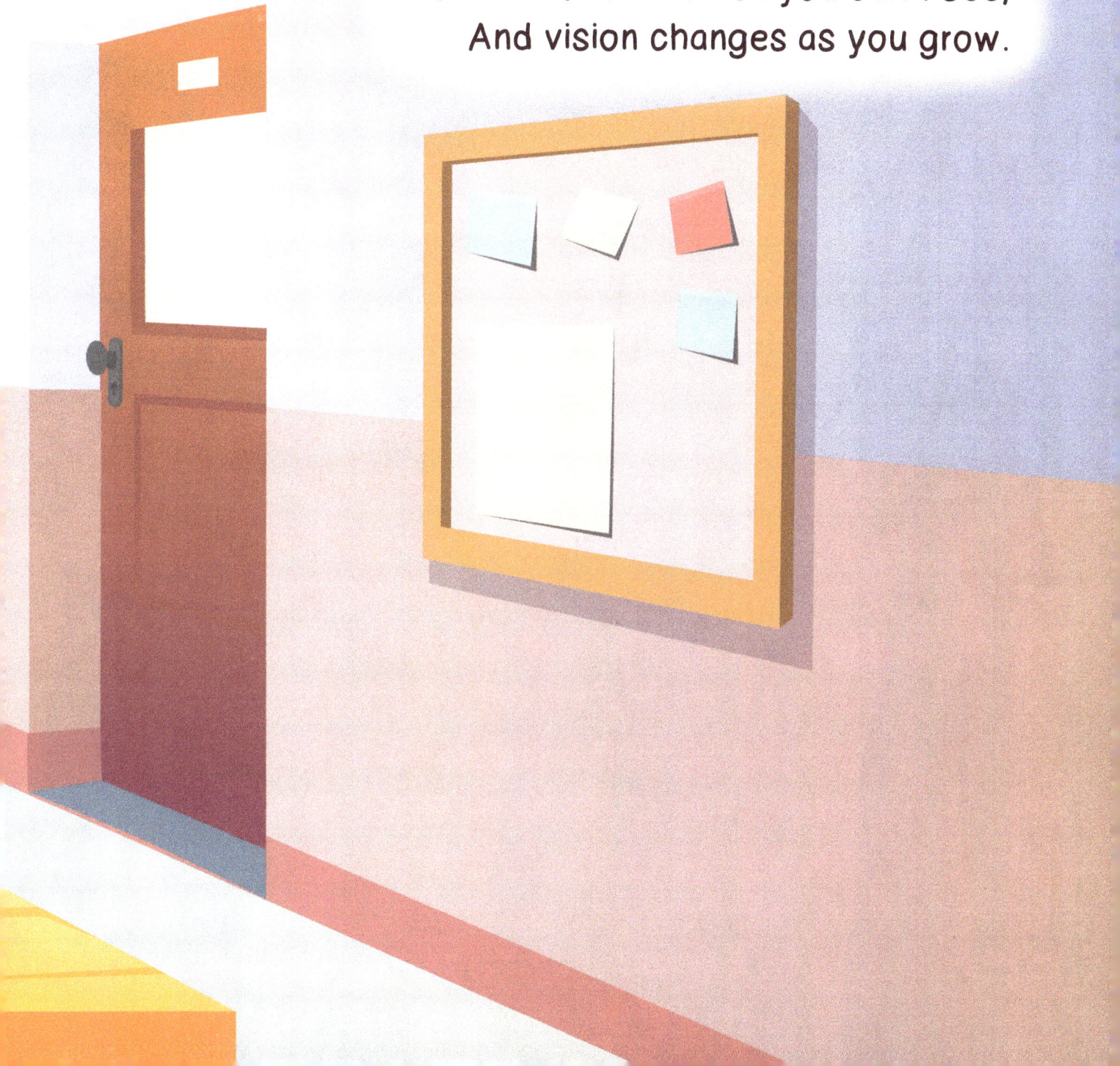

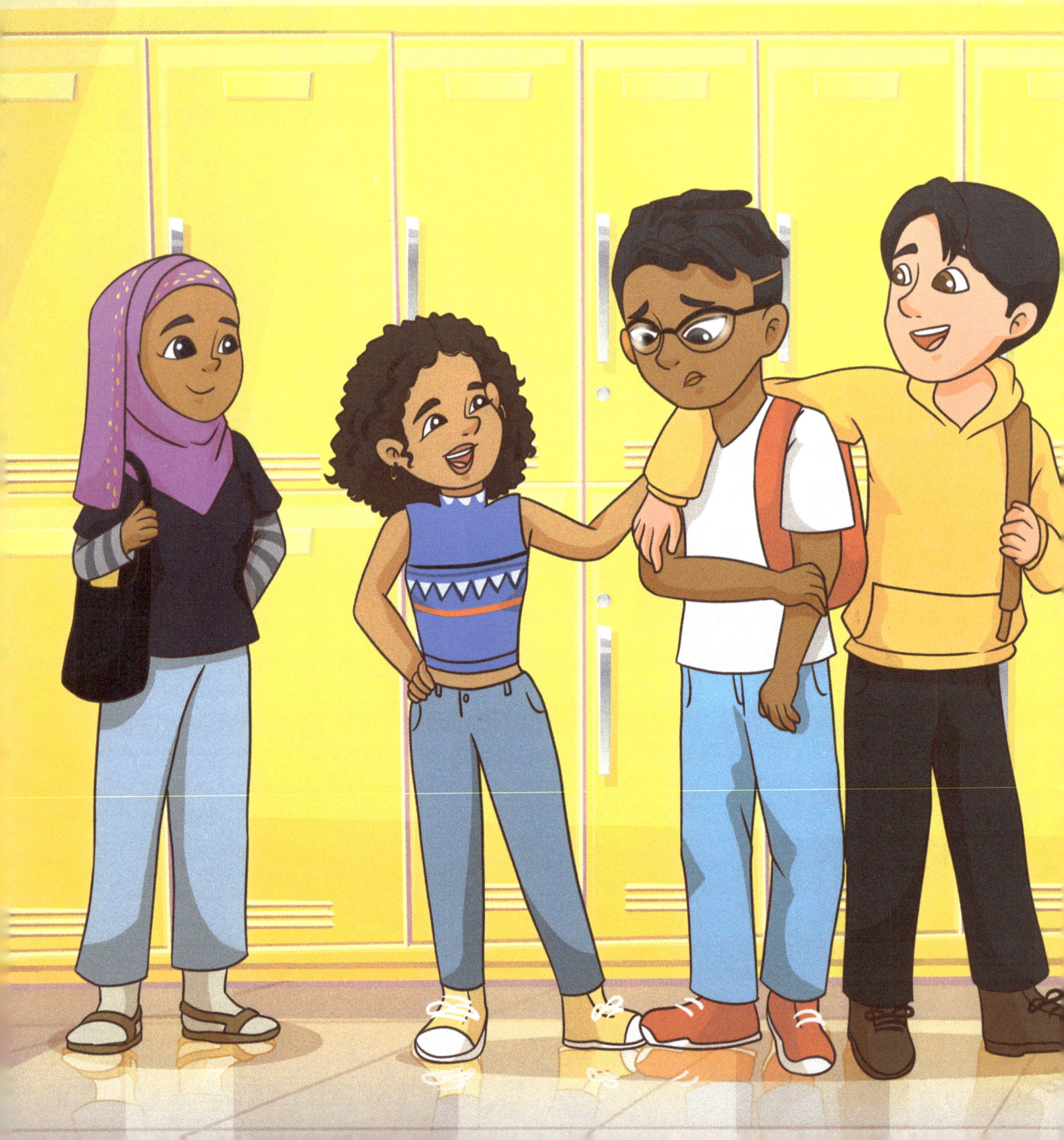

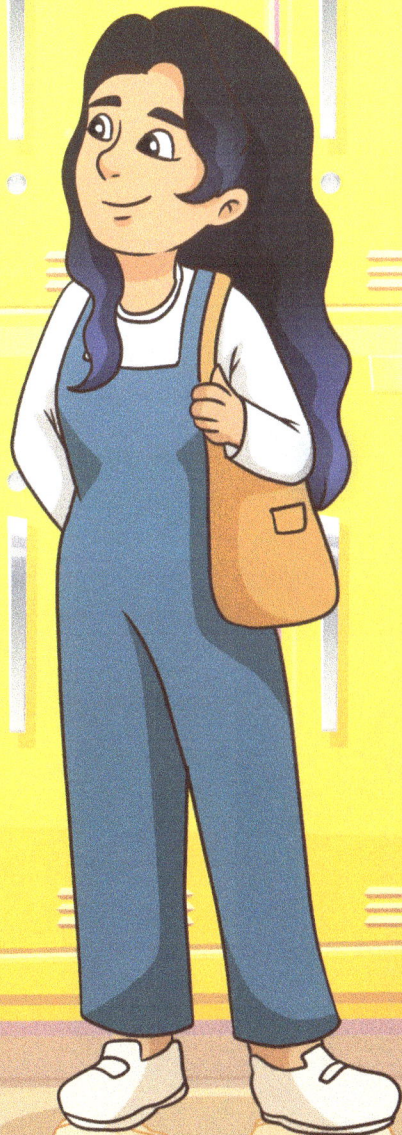

Why should I get an eye exam?
My friends might laugh at me.
They don't understand the value,
But glasses will help you to see.

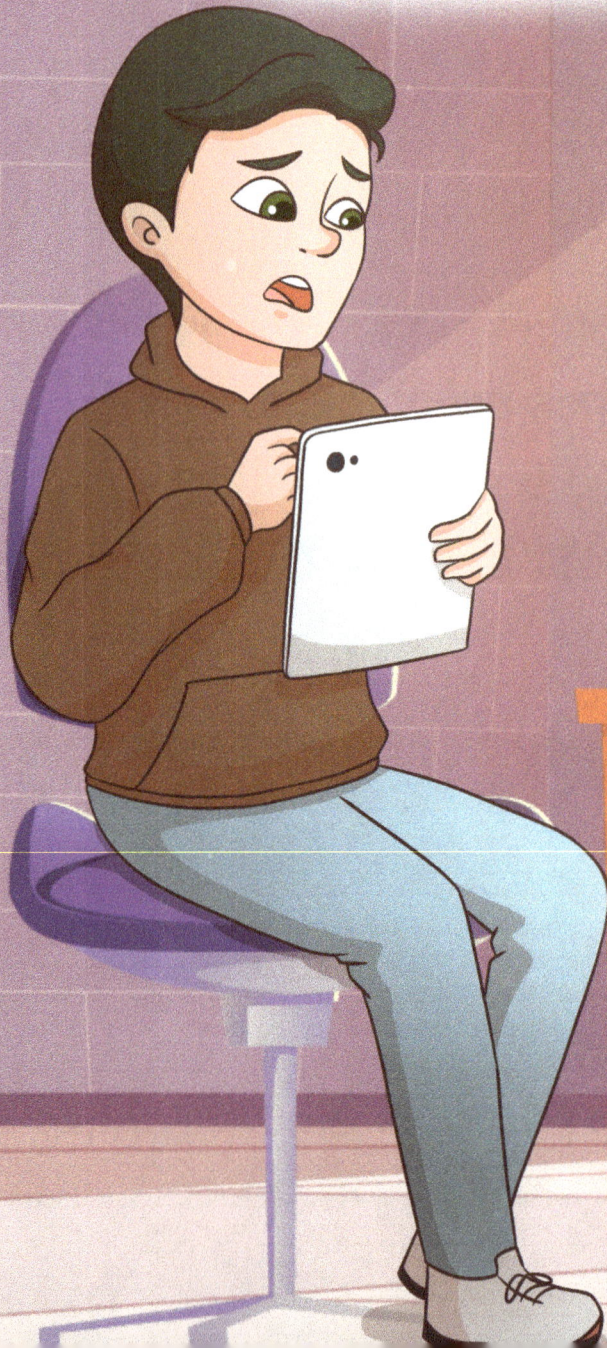

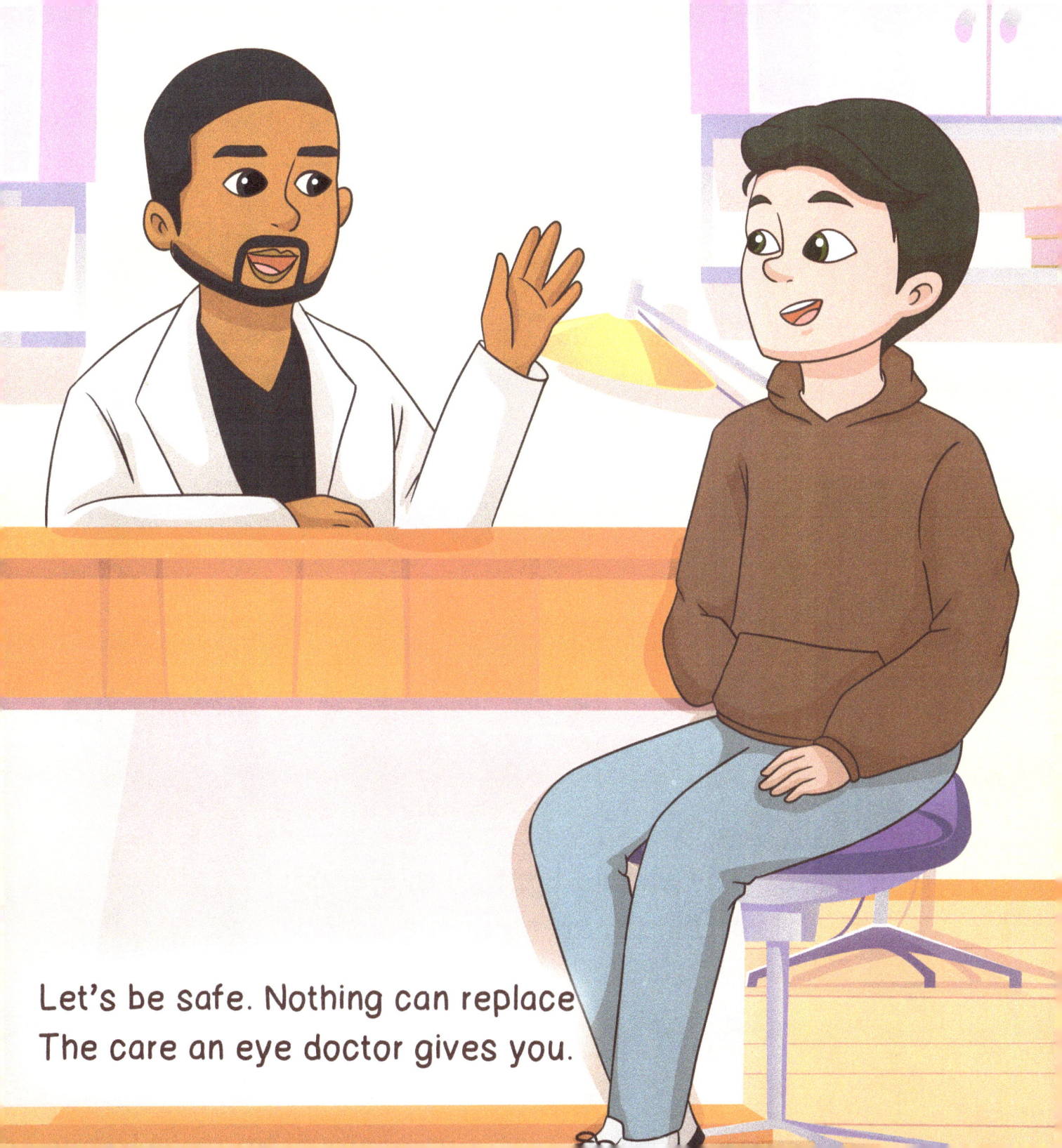

Let's be safe. Nothing can replace
The care an eye doctor gives you.

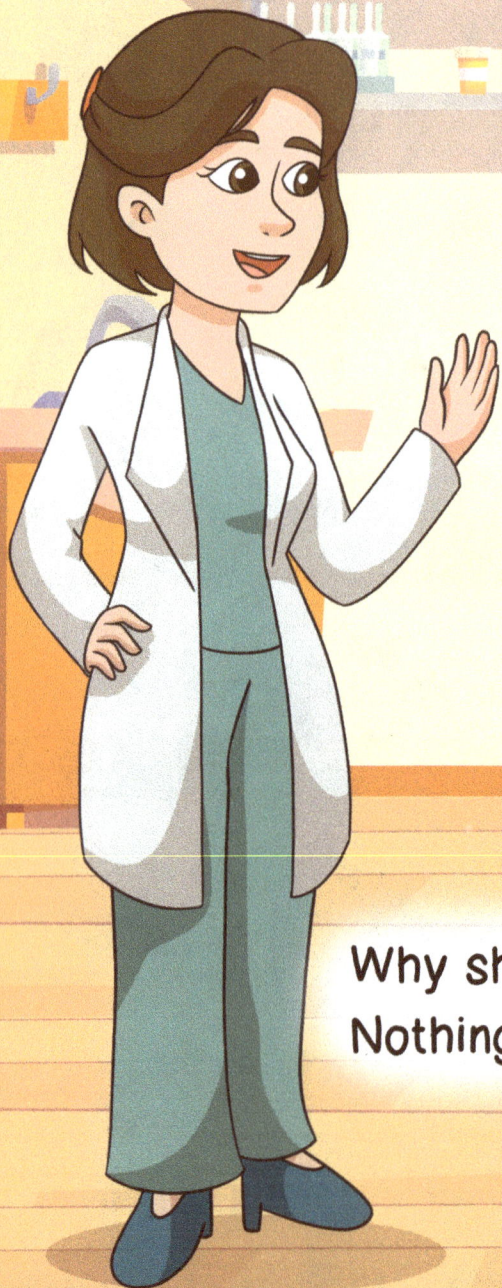

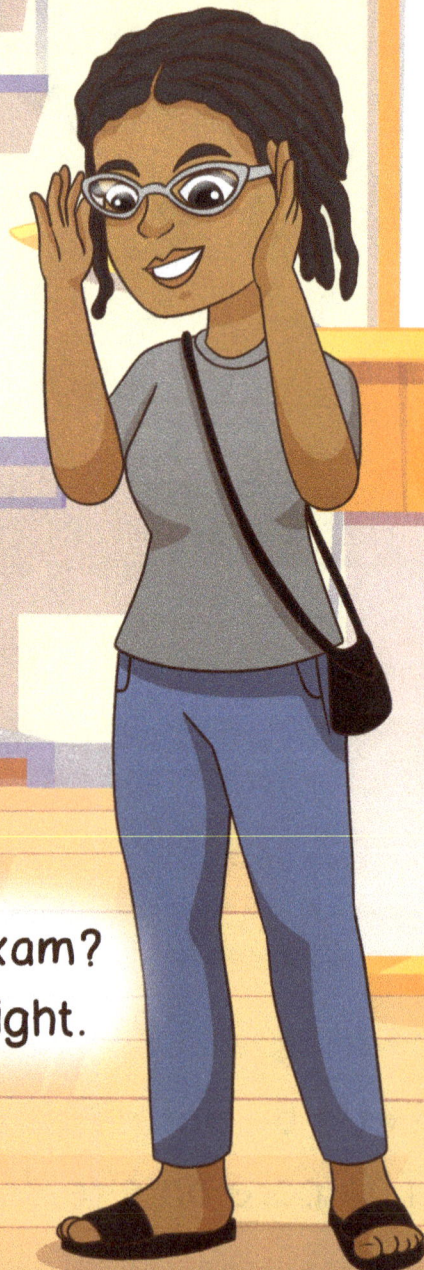

Why should I get an eye exam?
Nothing's wrong with my sight.

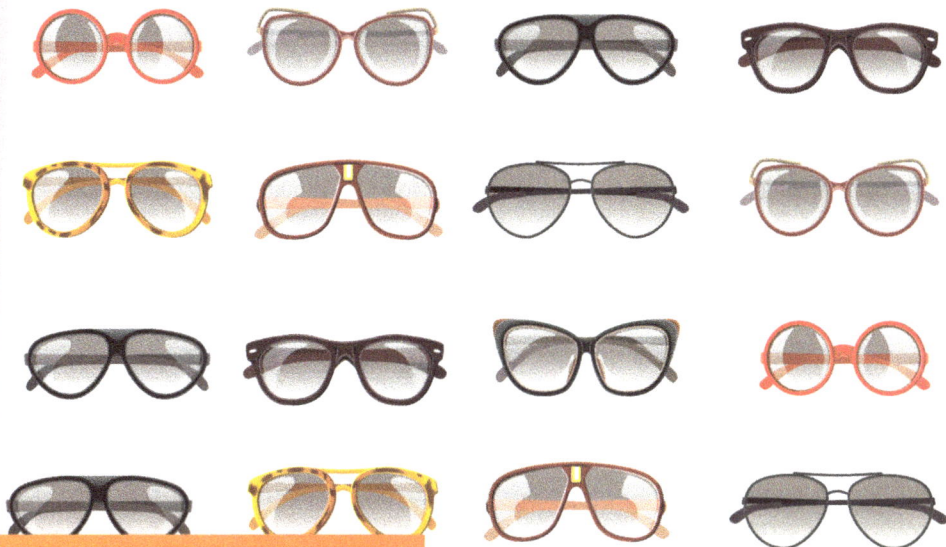

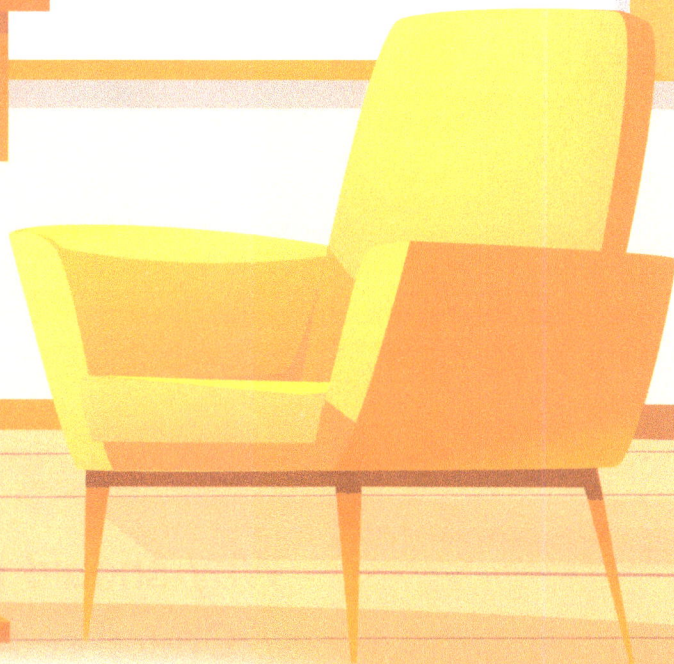

When you can't tell, your doctor can.
They know when things aren't right.

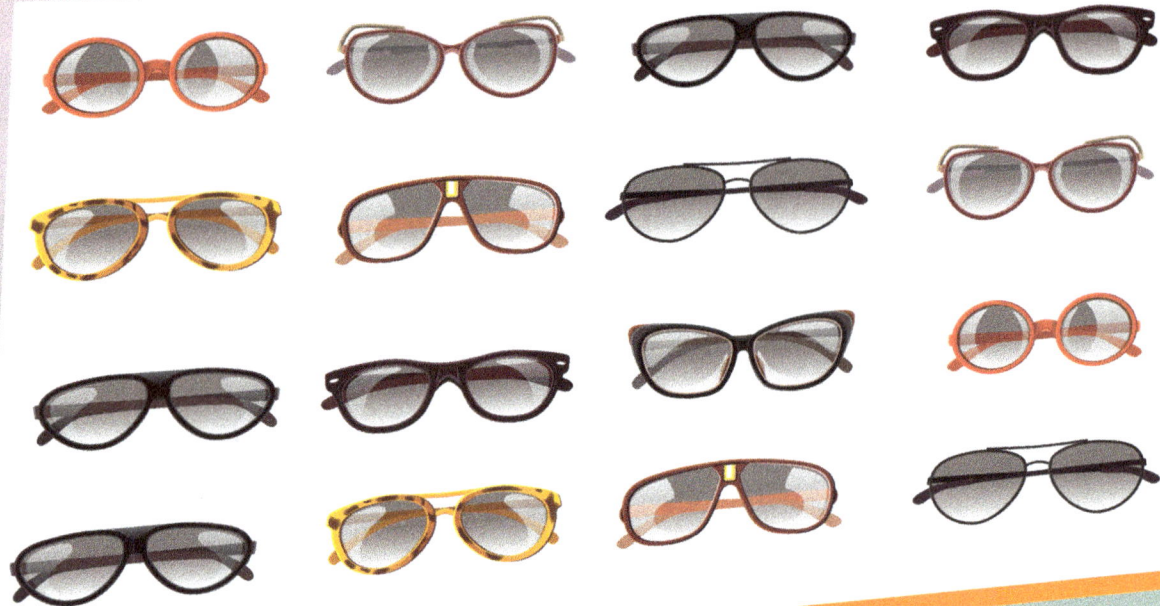

Why should I get an eye exam?
Cheap readers do just fine.
A custom pair and custom care
Will help you down the line.

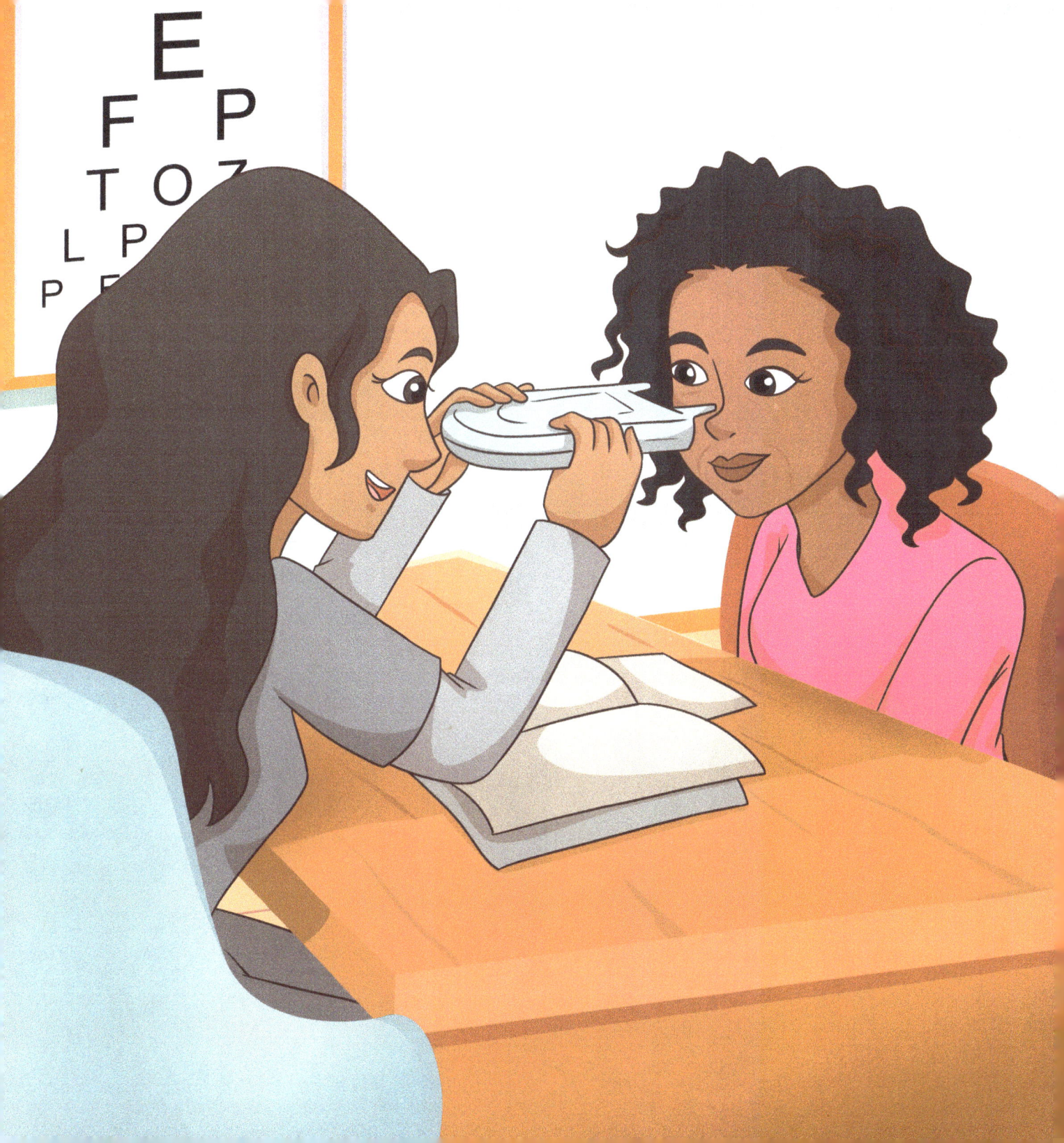

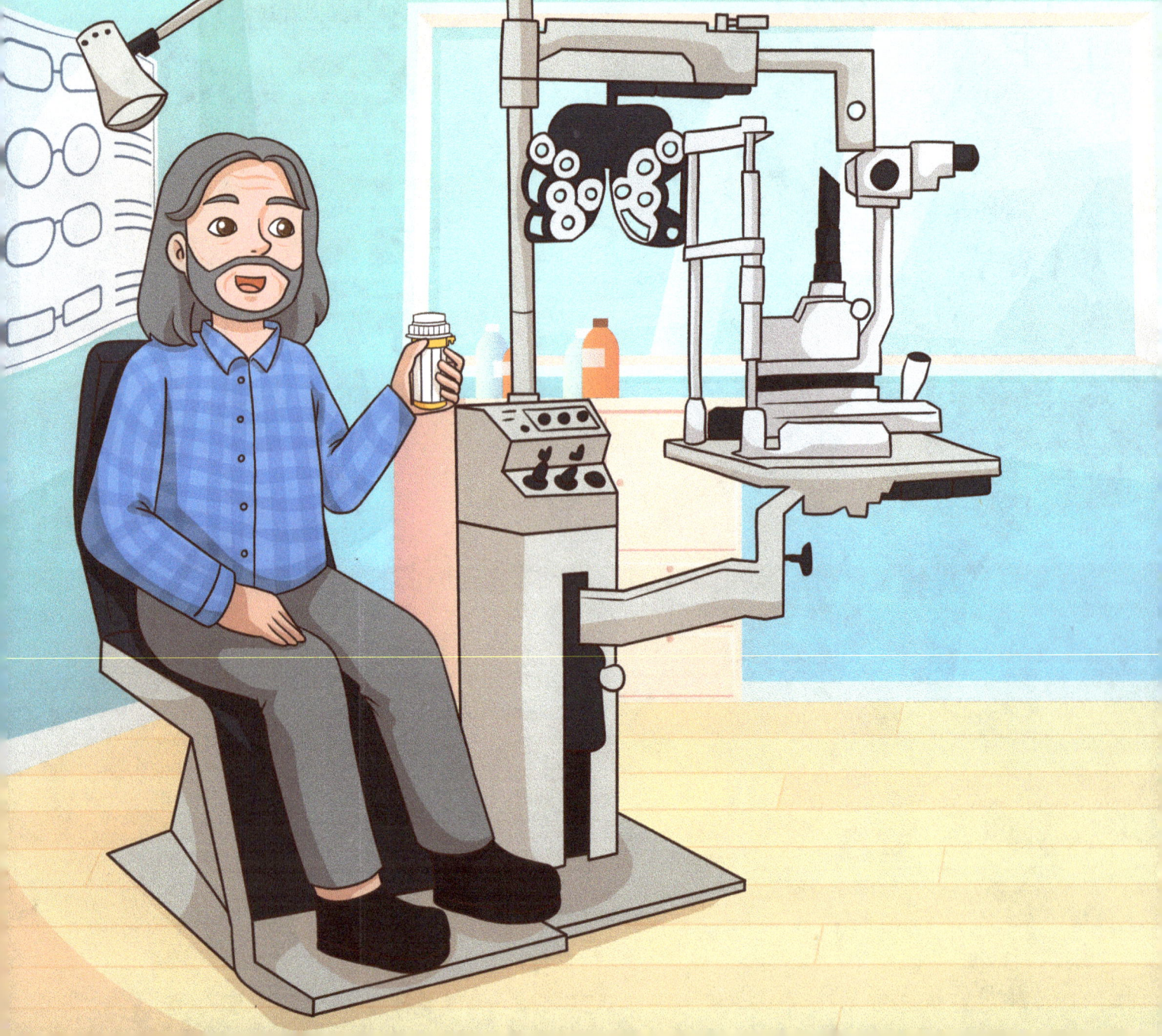

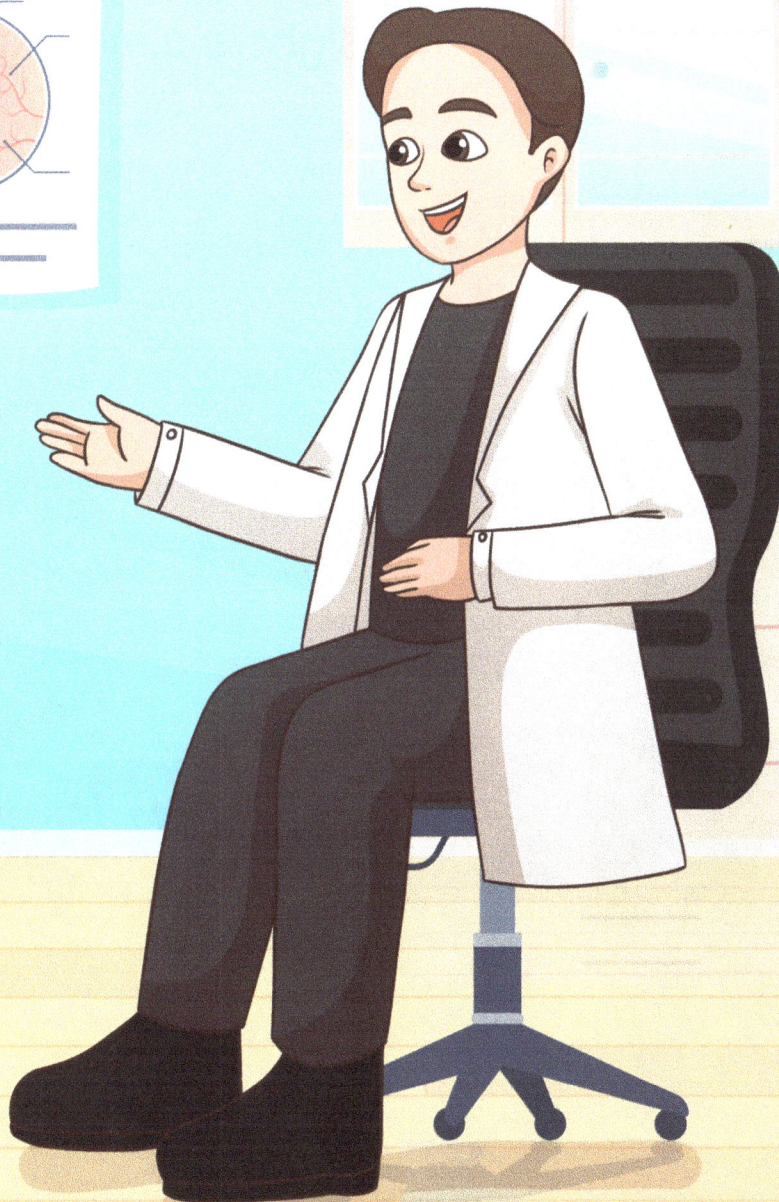

Why should I get an eye exam?
My sight is almost gone.

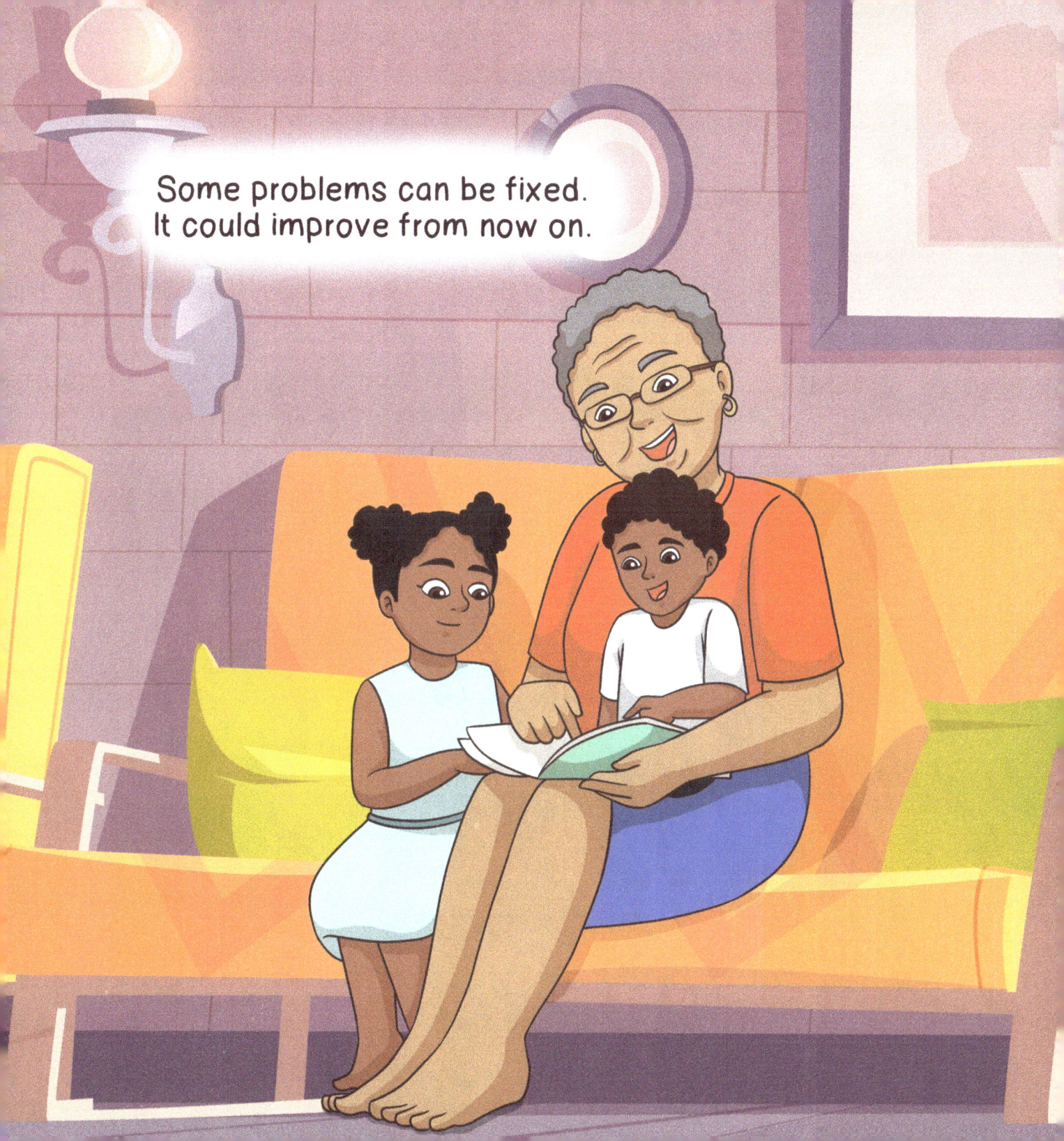

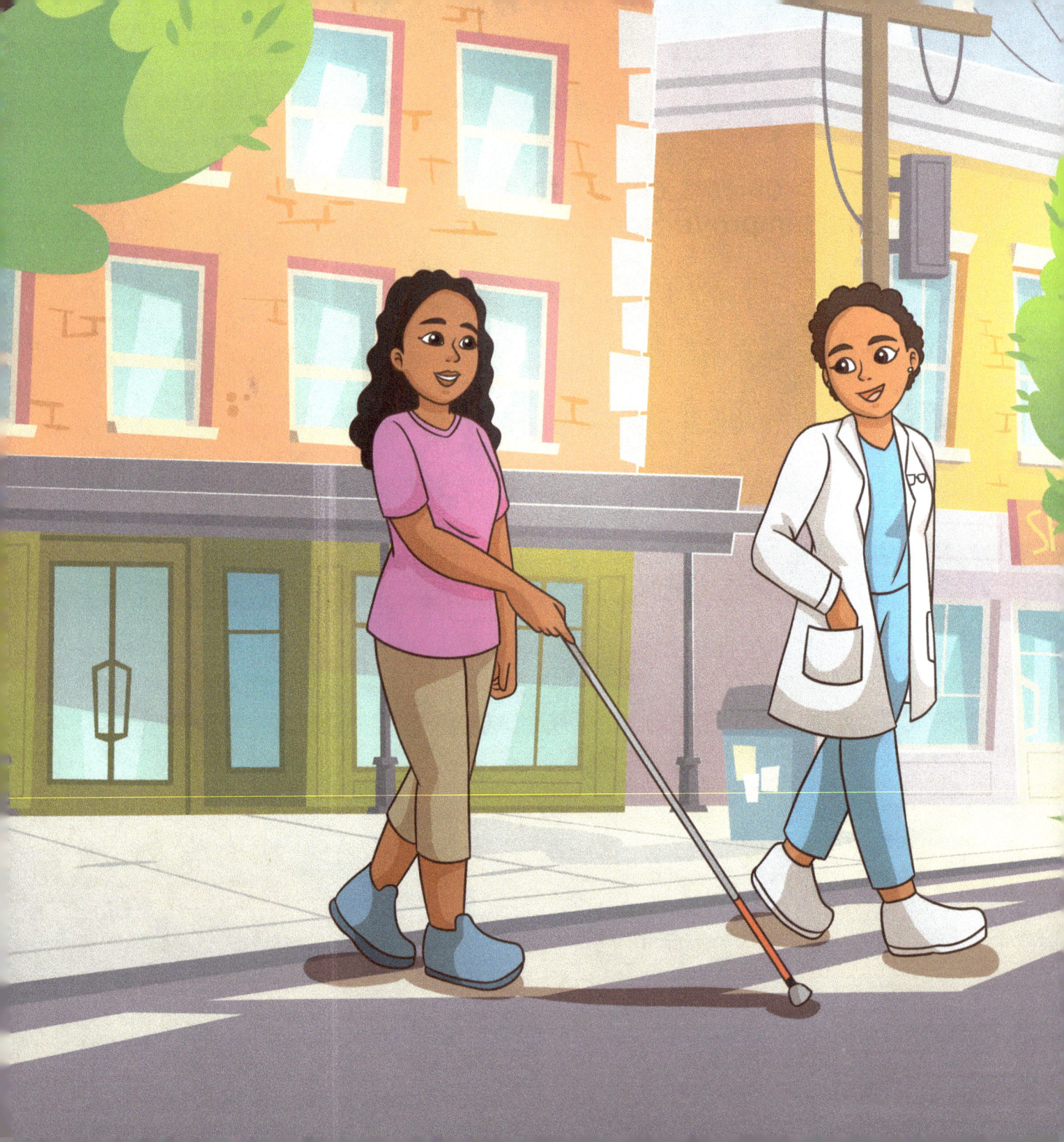

Why should I get an eye exam?
There is no hope for me.
Eye care is comprehensive,
And there's low vision therapy.

So... Why should you get an eye exam?
If you've made it through this list

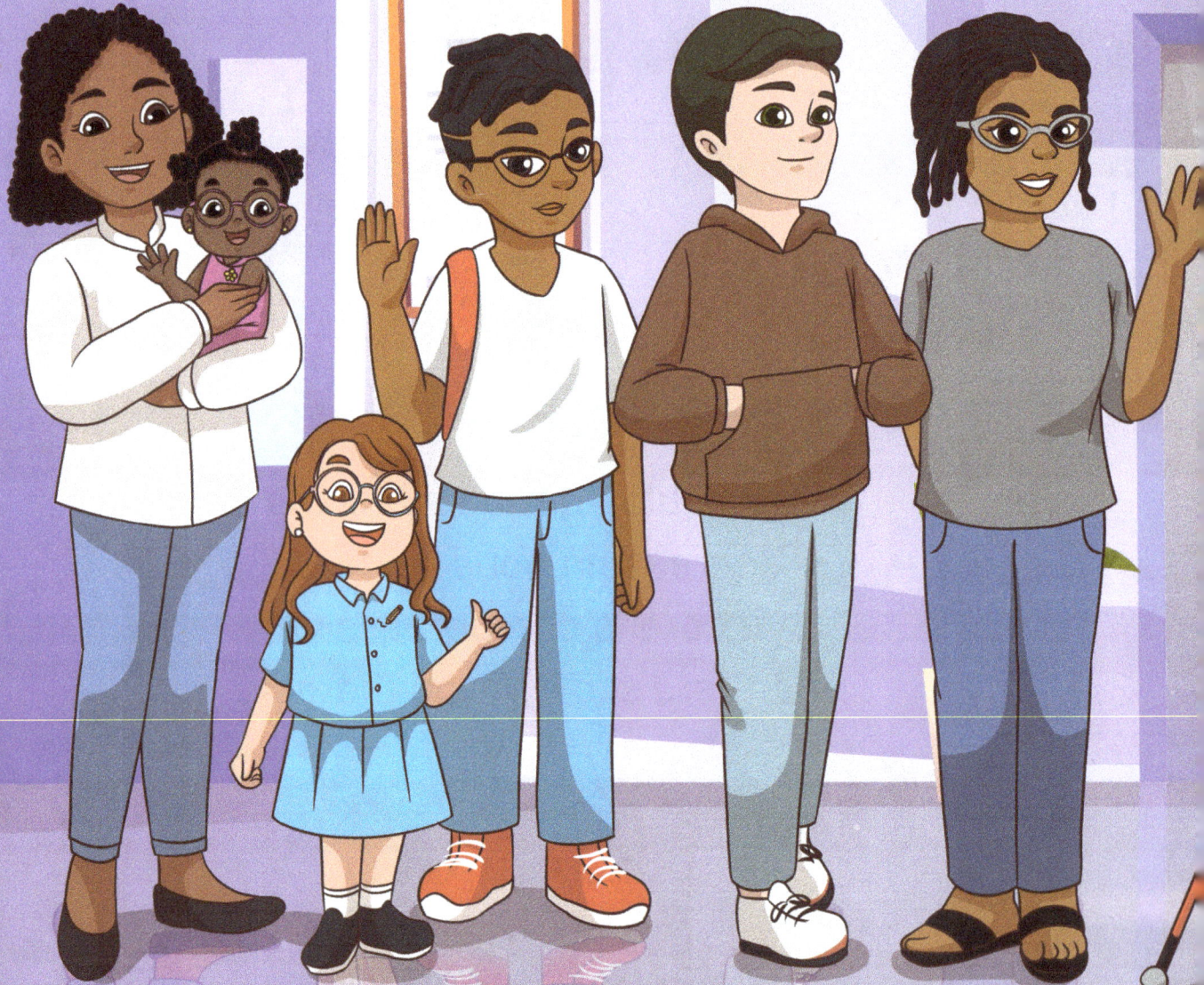

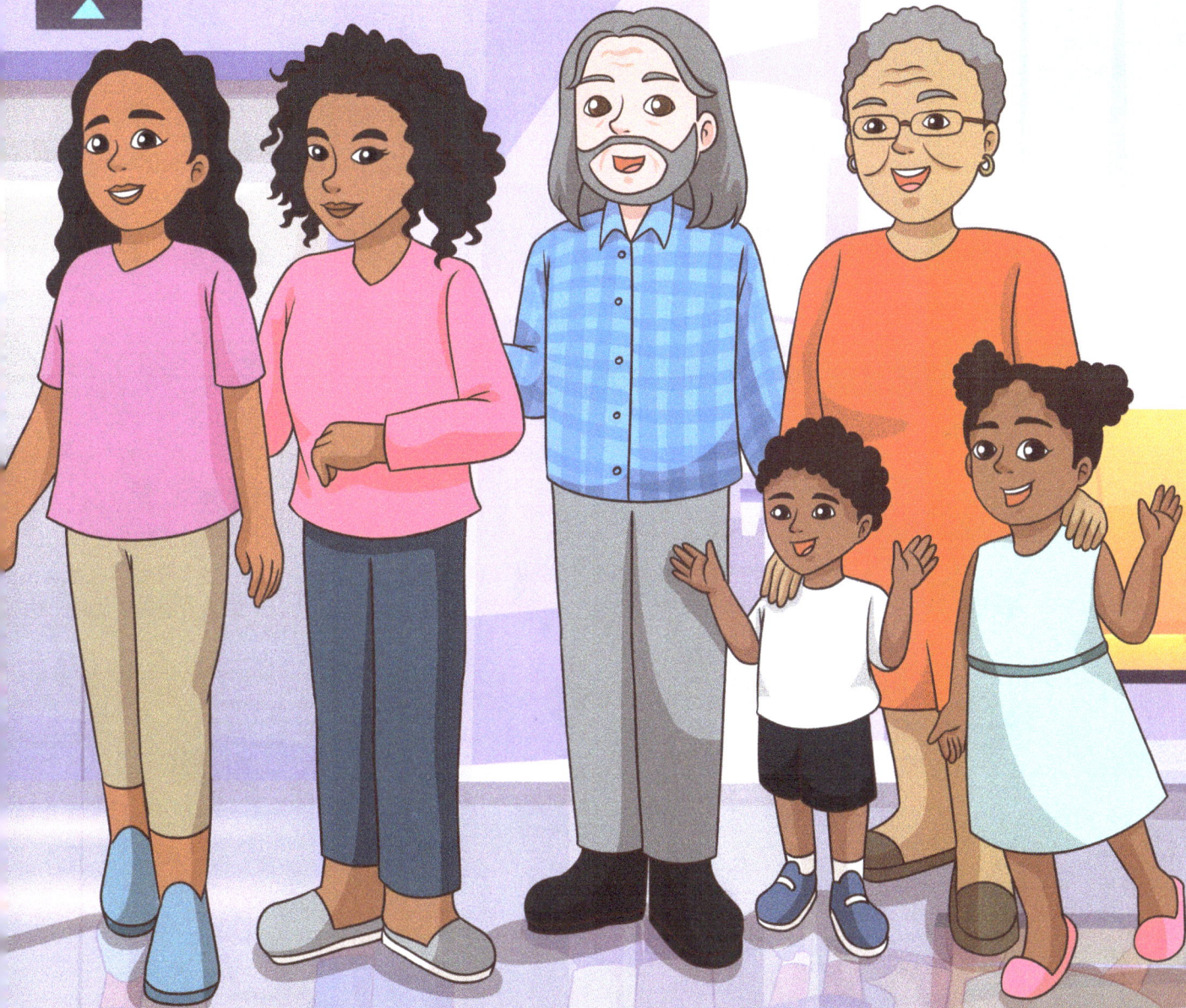

You know there are many reasons
To see an optometrist!

www.ingramcontent.com/pod-product-compliance
Lightning Source LLC
Chambersburg PA
CBHW080430030426
42335CB00020B/2663